SpringerBriefs in Statistics

For further volumes:
http://www.springer.com/series/8921

Ton J. Cleophas · Aeilko H. Zwinderman

Statistical Analysis of Clinical Data on a Pocket Calculator, Part 2

Statistics on a Pocket Calculator, Part 2

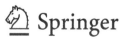 Springer

Ton J. Cleophas
Weresteijn 17
3363 BK Sliedrecht
The Netherlands

Aeilko H. Zwinderman
Rijnsburgerweg 54
2333 AC Leiden
The Netherlands

ISSN 2191-544X   ISSN 2191-5458 (electronic)
ISBN 978-94-007-4703-6 ISBN 978-94-007-4704-3 (eBook)
DOI 10.1007/978-94-007-4704-3
Springer Dordrecht Heidelberg New York London

Library of Congress Control Number: 2012939200

Printed on acid-free paper

Springer is part of Springer Science+Business Media (www.springer.com)

Preface

The small book "Statistical Analysis of Clinical Data on a Pocket Calculator" edited in 2011 presented 20 chapters of cookbook-like step-by-step analyses of clinical data, and was written for clinical investigators and medical students as a basic approach to the understanding and carrying out of medical statistics. It addressed the following subjects:

(1) statistical tests for continuous/binary data,
(2) power and samples size assessments,
(3) the calculation of confidence intervals,
(4) calculating variabilities,
(5) adjustments for multiple testing,
(6) reliability assessments of qualitative and quantitative diagnostic tests.

This book is a logical continuation and reviews additional pocket calculator methods that are important to data analysis, such as

(1) logarithmic and invert logarithmic transformations,
(2) binary partitioning,
(3) propensity score matching,
(4) mean and hot deck imputations,
(5) precision assessments of diagnostic tests,
(6) robust variabilities.

These methods are, generally, difficult on a statistical software program and easy on a pocket calculator. We should add that pocket calculators work faster, because summary statistics are used. Also, you understand better what you are doing. Pocket calculators are wonderful: they enable you to test instantly without the need to download a statistical software program.

The methods can also help you make use of methodologies for which there is little software, like Bhattacharya modeling, fuzzy models, Markov models, binary partitioning, etc.

We do hope that "Statistical Analysis of Clinical Data on a Pocket Calculator 1 and 2 " will enhance your understanding and carrying out of medical statistics, and help you dig deeper into the fascinating world of statistical data analysis. We recommend to those completing the current books, to study, as a next step, the two books entitled "SPSS for Starters 1 and 2" by the same authors.

Lyon, France, March 2012   Ton J. Cleophas
                                                                                 Aeilko H. Zwinderman

Contents

Chapter 1
Introduction

The first part of this title contained all of the statistical tests that are relevant to starting clinical investigators, and included statistical tests for continuous and binary data, as well as tests for power, sample size, multiple testing, variability, confounding, interaction, and reliability. Many more statistical methods can be carried out on a pocket calculator, and this small e book reviews the most important of them.

Some of the chapters in this e book review methods that can be used as an alternative and/or addition to standard methods in case of problems with the data, e.g., the problems of missing data (Chap. 3), manipulated data (Chap. 4), multiple confounders (Chap. 5), predictions beyond observations (Chap. 6), and uncertainty of diagnostic tests (Chap. 7), and the problems of outliers. For example, the Chaps. 8, 9, 10, 11 and 12 review respectively robust tests, non-linear modeling, fuzzy modeling, goodness of fit testing, and Bhattacharya models, that can be helpful with outliers and non-linear patterns in the data.

Other chapters review methods that can make more of your research than basic tests generally can e.g. the Chap. 13 on item response modeling, the Chap. 14 on superiority testing, and the Chap. 15 on variability testing. Binary partitioning for classification and regression tree (CART) methods are in Chap. 16. The basic principles of pooling the data in a meta-analysis, and testing for heterogeneity are reviewed in the Chaps. 17 and 18. Simple statistical tests for incident analysis and unexpected observations at the workplace are, finally, reviewed in the Chaps. 19 and 20.

Each test method is reported together with (1) a data example from practice, (2) all steps to be taken using a scientific pocket calculator, and (3) the main results and their interpretation. All of the methods described are fast, and can be correctly carried out on a scientific pocket calculator, such as the Casio fx-825, the Texas TI-30, the Sigma AK222, the Commodore and many other makes. Although several of the described methods can also be carried out with the help of statistical software, the latter procedure will be considerably slower.

T. J. Cleophas and A. H. Zwinderman, *Statistical Analysis of Clinical Data on a Pocket Calculator, Part 2*, SpringerBriefs in Statistics, DOI: 10.1007/978-94-007-4704-3_1, © The Author(s) 2012

In order to obtain a better overview of the different test methods each chapter will start on an uneven page. Both part 1 and 2 of this issue will be applied as a major help to the workshops "Designing and performing clinical research" organized by the teaching department of Albert Schweitzer STZ (collaborative top clinical) Hospital Dordrecht, and the statistics modules at the European College of Pharmaceutical Medicine, Claude Bernard University, Lyon, and Academic Medical Center, Amsterdam.

The authors of this book are aware that it consists of a minimum of text and do hope that this will enhance the process of mastering the methods. Yet we recommend that for a better understanding of the test procedures the book be used together with the same authors' textbook "Statistics Applied to Clinical Studies" 5th edition edited 2012, by Springer Dordrecht Netherlands. More complex data files like data files with multiple treatment modalities or multiple predictor variables can not be analyzed with a pocket calculator. We recommend that the small books "SPSS for Starters," Parts 1 and 2 (Springer, Dordrecht, 2010, and 2012) from the same authors be used as a complementary help for the readers' benefit.

Chapter 2
Basic Logarithm for a Better Understanding of Statistical Methods

Non-linear relationships in clinical research are often linear after logarithmic transformations. Also, logarithmic transformation normalizes skewed frequency distributions and is used for the analysis of likelihood ratios. Basic knowledge of logarithms is, therefore, convenient for a better understanding of many statistical methods. Almost always natural logarithm (ln), otherwise called naperian logarithm, is used, i.e., logarithm to the base e. Log is logarithm to the base 10, ln is logarithm to the base e (2.718281828).

Theory and Basic Steps

$\log 10 = 10 \log 10 = 1$
$\log 100 = 10 \log 100 = 2$
$\log 1 = 10 \log 1 = 0$
antilog $1 = 10$
antilog $2 = 100$
antilog $0 = 1$

Casio fx-825 scientific, Scientific Calculator, Texas TI-30XA, Sigma, Commodore
Press: 100….log….2
Press: 2….2ndf….log…100

Electronic Calculator, Kenko KK-82MS-5
Press: 100…. = ….log…. = ….2
Press: 2…. = ….shift….log….100

$\ln e = e \log e = 1$
$\ln e^2 = e \log e^2 = 2$
$\ln 1 = e \log 1 = 0$

T. J. Cleophas and A. H. Zwinderman, *Statistical Analysis of Clinical Data on a Pocket Calculator, Part 2*, SpringerBriefs in Statistics, DOI: 10.1007/978-94-007-4704-3_2,

antiln $1 = 2.718...$
antiln $2 = 7.389...$
antiln $0 = 1$

Casio fx-825 scientific, Scientific Calculator, Texas TI-30XA, Sigma
Press: 7.389....ln....2
Press: 2....2ndf....ln....7389

Electronic Calculator, Kenko KK-82MS-5
Press: 7.389.... = ...ln.... = ...2
Press: 2.... = ...shift....ln....7.389

Example, Markov Model

In patients with diabetes mellitus (* = sign of multiplication):

After		
	1 year 10% has beta-cell failure, and	90% has not.
	2	90 * 90 = 81% has not.
	3	90 * 90 * 90 = 73% has not.

When will 50% have beta-cell failure?

$0.9^x = 0.5$
x log 0.9 = log 0.5
x = log 0.5/log 0.9 = 6.5788 years.

Example, Odds Ratios

	Events	No events	
	Numbers of patients		
Group 1	15(a)	20(b)	35(a + b)
Group 2	15(c)	5(d)	20(c + d)
	30(a + c)	25(b + d)	55(a + b + c + d)

The odds of an event = the number of patients in a group with an event divided by the number without. In group 1 the odds of an event equals = a/b.
The odds ratio (OR) of group 1 compared to group 2

$$= (a/b)/(c/d)$$
$$= (15/20)/(15/5)$$
$$= 0.25$$

lnOR　　$= \ln 0.25 = -1.386(\ln = $ natural logarithm$)$

The standard error (SE) of the above term

$$= \sqrt{(1/\,a\,+1/\,b\,+1/\,c\,+1/\,d)}$$
$$= \sqrt{(1/15 + 1/20 + 1/15 + 1/5)}$$
$$= \sqrt{0.38333}$$
$$= 0.619$$

The odds ratio can be tested using the z-test.

$$\text{The test} - \text{statistic} = \text{z} - \text{value}$$
$$= (\ln \text{odds ratio}) / (\text{SE } \ln \text{odds ratio})$$
$$= -1.386/0.619$$
$$= -2.239$$

Z table

	Z-value	P-value
	1.645	0.1
	1.960	0.05
	2.5576	0.01
	3.090	0.002

The z table shows that if this value is smaller than -1.96 or larger than $+1.96$, then the odds ratio is significantly different from 1 with p-value $<.05$. There is, thus, a significant difference in numbers of events between the two groups.

Conclusion

We conclude that basic knowledge of logarithms is convenient for a better understanding of many statistical methods. Odds ratio tests, log likelihood ratio tests, Markov modeling and many regression models use logarithmic transformations.

Chapter 3
Missing Data Imputation

Missing data in clinical research data is often a real problem. As an example, a 35 patient data file of three variables consists of $3 \times 35 = 105$ values if the data are complete. With only five values missing (one value missing per patient) five patients will not have complete data, and are rather useless for the analysis. This is not 5 % but 15 % of this small study population of 35 patients. An analysis of the remaining 85 % patients is likely not to be powerful to demonstrate the effects we wished to assess. This illustrates the necessity of data imputation.

Four methods of data imputation are available; (1) mean imputation, (2) hot deck imputation, (3) regression imputation, (4) multiple imputations. In the current chapter the methods (1) and (2) will be given. In the book SPSS for Starters Part 2 (Cleophas and Zwinderman, (ed) Springer New York, 2012, Chap. 12) the methods (3) and (4) will be given.

A condition for any type of data imputation is that the missing data are not clustered but randomly distributed in the data file. An example is in the table on the next page.

The table on the page 9 gives the results of mean imputation of these data. The missing values are imputed by the mean values of the different variables. The table on the page 10 gives the results of hot deck imputation. The missing data are imputed by those of the closest neighbor observed: the missing value is imputed with the value of an individual whose non-missing data are closest to those of the patient with the missing value. Imputed data are of course not real data, but constructed values that should increase the sensitivity of testing. Regression imputation is more sensitive than mean and hot deck imputation, but it often overstates sensitivity. Probably, the best method for data imputation is multiple imputations (4), because this method works as a device for representing missing data uncertainty.

T. J. Cleophas and A. H. Zwinderman, *Statistical Analysis of Clinical Data on a Pocket Calculator, Part 2*, SpringerBriefs in Statistics, DOI: 10.1007/978-94-007-4704-3_3, © The Author(s) 2012

Table data file with random missing data (lax = laxative)

New lax	Bisacodyl	Age
24,00	8,00	25,00
30,00	13,00	30,00
25,00	15,00	25,00
35,00	10,00	31,00
39,00	9,00	
30,00	10,00	33,00
27,00	8,00	22,00
14,00	5,00	18,00
39,00	13,00	14,00
42,00		30,00
41,00	11,00	36,00
38,00	11,00	30,00
39,00	12,00	27,00
37,00	10,00	38,00
47,00	18,00	40,00
	13,00	31,00
36,00	12,00	25,00
12,00	4,00	24,00
26,00	10,00	27,00
20,00	8,00	20,00
43,00	16,00	35,00
31,00	15,00	29,00
40,00	14,00	32,00
31,00		30,00
36,00	12,00	40,00
21,00	6,00	31,00
44,00	19,00	41,00
11,00	5,00	26,00
27,00	8,00	24,00
24,00	9,00	30,00
40,00	15,00	
32,00	7,00	31,00
10,00	6,00	23,00
37,00	14,00	43,00
19,00	7,00	30,00

Mean values of the variable are imputated in the missing data from the above table (the imputed data are in underlined, lax = laxative)

New lax	Bisacodyl	Age
24,00	8,00	25,00
30,00	13,00	30,00
25,00	15,00	25,00
35,00	10,00	31,00

(continued)

(continued)

Mean values of the variable are imputated in the missing data from the above table (the imputed data are in underlined, lax = laxative)

New lax	Bisacodyl	Age
39,00	9,00	29,00
30,00	10,00	33,00
27,00	8,00	22,00
14,00	5,00	18,00
39,00	13,00	14,00
42,00	11,00	30,00
41,00	11,00	36,00
38,00	11,00	30,00
39,00	12,00	27,00
37,00	10,00	38,00
47,00	18,00	40,00
30,00	13,00	31,00
36,00	12,00	25,00
12,00	4,00	24,00
26,00	10,00	27,00
20,00	8,00	20,00
43,00	16,00	35,00
31,00	15,00	29,00
40,00	14,00	32,00
31,00	11,00	30,00
36,00	12,00	40,00
21,00	6,00	31,00
44,00	19,00	41,00
11,00	5,00	26,00
27,00	8,00	24,00
24,00	9,00	30,00
40,00	15,00	29,00
32,00	7,00	31,00
10,00	6,00	23,00
37,00	14,00	43,00
19,00	7,00	30,00

The closest neighbor data were imputed in the missing data from the above table (lax = laxative)

New lax	Bisacodyl	Age
24,00	8,00	25,00
30,00	13,00	30,00
25,00	15,00	25,00
35,00	10,00	31,00
39,00	9,00	30,00
30,00	10,00	33,00
27,00	8,00	22,00

(continued)

(continued)

The closest neighbor data were imputed in the missing data from the above table (lax = laxative)

New lax	Bisacodyl	Age
14,00	5,00	18,00
39,00	13,00	14,00
42,00	14,00	30,00
41,00	11,00	36,00
38,00	11,00	30,00
39,00	12,00	27,00
37,00	10,00	38,00
47,00	18,00	40,00
30,00	13,00	31,00
36,00	12,00	25,00
12,00	4,00	24,00
26,00	10,00	27,00
20,00	8,00	20,00
43,00	16,00	35,00
31,00	15,00	29,00
40,00	14,00	32,00
31,00	15,00	30,00
36,00	12,00	40,00
21,00	6,00	31,00
44,00	19,00	41,00
11,00	5,00	26,00
27,00	8,00	24,00
24,00	9,00	30,00
40,00	15,00	32,00
32,00	7,00	31,00
10,00	6,00	23,00
37,00	14,00	43,00
19,00	7,00	30,00

Conclusion

Missing data in clinical research is often a real problem. Mean and hot deck imputation produces constructed values that should increase the sensitivity of testing.

Chapter 4
Assessing Manipulated Data

Statistics is not good at detecting manipulated data, but it can assess the consistence of the data with randomness. An example is given of a cholesterol reducing trial. The results consisted of 96 risk ratios, and often a 0, 1 or 9 was observed as final digit of the odds ratios, while the values 2–8 as final digits were virtually unobserved. We will test whether the observed frequencies of the final digits are compatible with equal frequencies, as expected, and we will use a Chi-square test for that purpose.

Final digit of RR	Observed frequency	Expected frequency	$\Sigma(\text{observed}-\text{expected})^2/\text{expected}$
0	23	9.6	18.7
1	40	9.6	96.3
2	3	9.6	4.5
3	0	9.6	9.6
4	0	9.6	9.6
5	0	9.6	9.6
6	0	9.6	9.6
7	1	9.6	7.7
8	3	9.6	4.5
9	26	9.6	28.0
Total	96	96.0	198.1

The Chi-square-value for $9-1 = 8$ degrees of freedom equals 198.1. According to the Chi-square table (see next page), this is much larger than 26.124. This mean that the difference between observed and expected is much larger than could happen by chance with a p-value <0.001. The conclusion should be that the final digits are not random, and that the validity of this study is in jeopardy.

T. J. Cleophas and A. H. Zwinderman, *Statistical Analysis of Clinical Data on a Pocket Calculator, Part 2*, SpringerBriefs in Statistics, DOI: 10.1007/978-94-007-4704-3_4,
© The Author(s) 2012

Chi-Square Table (X² - Table)

The underneath Chi-square table (χ^2-table) gives columns and rows: the upper row gives the p-values. The first column gives the degrees of freedom which adjust for sample size (or numbers of cells in a cross-tab). With 8 degrees of freedom look at the 8th row. Our calculated chi-square value is much larger than all of the values in the row. The p-value is thus much smaller than 0.001. This means that that the final digits are much more different from expected than could happen by chance.

Chi-squared distribution

Two-tailed p-value

df	0.10	0.05	0.01	0.001
1	2.706	3.841	6.635	10.827
2	4.605	5.991	9.210	13.815
3	6.251	7.815	11.345	16.266
4	7.779	9.488	13.277	18.466
5	9.236	11.070	15.086	20.515
6	10.645	12.592	16.812	22.457
7	12.017	14.067	18.475	24.321
8	13.362	15.507	20.090	26.124
9	14.684	16.919	21.666	27.877
10	15.987	18.307	23.209	29.588
11	17.275	19.675	24.725	31.264
12	18.549	21.026	26.217	32.909
13	19.812	22.362	27.688	34.527
14	21.064	23.685	29.141	36.124
15	22.307	24.996	30.578	37.698
16	23.542	26.296	32.000	39.252
17	24.769	27.587	33.409	40.791
18	25.989	28.869	31.805	42.312
19	27.204	30.144	36.191	43.819
20	28.412	31.410	37.566	45.314
21	29.615	32.671	38.932	46.796
22	30.813	33.924	40.289	48.268
23	32.007	35.172	41.638	49.728
24	33.196	36.415	42.980	51.179
25	34.382	37.652	44.314	52.619
26	35.563	38.885	45.642	54.051
27	36.741	40.113	46.963	55.475
28	37.916	41.337	48.278	56.892
29	39.087	42.557	49.588	58.301
30	40.256	43.773	50.892	59.702
40	51.805	55.758	63.691	73.403
50	63.167	67.505	76.154	86.660

(continued)

(continued)

Two-tailed p-value

df	0.10	0.05	0.01	0.001
60	74.397	79.082	88.379	99.608
70	85.527	90.531	100.43	112.32
80	96.578	101.88	112.33	124.84
90	107.57	113.15	124.12	137.21
100	118.50	124.34	135.81	149.45

Conclusion

Statistics is not good at detecting manipulated data, but it can assess the consistence of the data with randomness. The final digit method is convenient for the purpose.

Chapter 5
Propensity Scores and Propensity Score Matching for Assessing Multiple Confounders

Propensity score are ideal for assessing confounding, particularly, if multiple confounders are in a study. E.g., age and cardiovascular risk factors may not be similarly distributed in two treatment groups of a parallel-group study. Propensity score matching is used to make observational data look like randomized controlled trial data.

Propensity Scores

A propensity score for age can be defined as the risk ratio (or rather odds ratio) of receiving treatment 1 compared to that of treatment 2 if you are old in this study.

		Treatment-1 n = 100	Treatment-2 n = 100	Odds treatment-1/odds treatment-2 (OR)
1.	Age >65	63	76	0.54(63/76 /37/24)
2.	Age <65	37	24	1.85(= OR_2 =1/OR_1)
3.	Diabetes	20	33	0.51
4.	Not diabetes	80	67	1.96
5.	Smoker	50	80	0.25
6.	Not smoker	50	20	4.00
7.	Hypertension	51	65	0.65
8.	Not hypertension	49	35	1.78
9.	Not cholesterol	39	22	2.27

The odds ratios can be tested for statistical significance (see Chap. 2, odds ratios), and those that are statistically significant can, then, be used for calculating a combined propensity-score for all of the inequal characteristics by multiplying

T. J. Cleophas and A. H. Zwinderman, *Statistical Analysis of Clinical Data on a Pocket Calculator, Part 2*, SpringerBriefs in Statistics, DOI: 10.1007/978-94-007-4704-3_5,

the significant odds ratios, and, then, calculating from this product the combined propensity-score = combined "risk ratio" (= combined OR/(1+ combined OR). y = yes, n = no, combined OR = $OR_1 \times OR_3 \times OR_5 \times OR_7 \times OR_9$

	Old	diab	smoker	Hypert	Cholesterol	Combined OR	Combined propensity score
Patient 1	y	n	n	y	y	7.99	0.889
2	n	n	n	y	y	105.27	0.991
3	y	n	n	y	y	22.80	0.958
4	y	y	y	y	y	0.4999	0.333
5	n	n	y				
6	y	y	y				
7	.....						
8	....						

Each patient has his/her own propensity score based on and adjusted for the significantly larger chance of receiving one treatment versus the other treatment.

Usually, propensity score adjustment for confounders is accomplished by dividing the patients into four subgroups, but for the purpose of simplicity we here use 2 subgroups, those with high and those with low propensity scores.

Confounding is assessed by the method of subclassification. In the above example an overall mean difference between the two treatment modalities is calculated.

For treatment zero
Mean effect ± standard error (SE) = 1.5 units ± 0.5 units
For treatment one
Mean effect ± SE = 2.5 units ± 0.6 units

The mean difference of the two treatments

$$= 1.0 \text{ units } \pm \text{ pooled standard error pooled standard error}$$
$$= 1.0 \pm \sqrt{(0.5^2 + 0.6^2)}$$
$$= 1.0 \pm 0.61$$

The t - value as calculated $= 1.0/0.61 = 1.639$

With $100-2$ (100 patients, 2 groups) = 98 degrees of freedom the p-value of this difference is calculated to be

$$= p > 0.10 \text{ (according to t - table at the end of this chapter)}.$$

In order to assess the possibility of confounding, a weighted mean has to be calculated. The underneath equation is adequate for the purpose (prop score = propensity score).

$$\text{Weighted mean} = \frac{\text{Difference}_{\text{high prop score}}/\text{ its SE}^2 + \text{Difference}_{\text{low prop score}}/\text{ its SE}^2}{1/\text{ SE}^2_{\text{high prop score}} + 1/\text{ SE}^2_{\text{low prop score}}}$$

For the high prop score we find means of 2.0 and 3.0 units, for the low prop score 1.0 and 2.0 units. The mean difference separately are 1.0 and 1.0 as expected. However, the pooled standard errors are different, for the males 0.4, and for the females 0.3 units.

According to the above equation a weighted t-value is calculated

$$\text{Weighted mean} = \frac{(1.0/0.4^2 + 1.0/0.3^2)}{(1/0.4^2 + 1/0.3^2)}$$

$$= 1.0$$

$$\text{Weighted SE}^2 = \frac{1}{(1/0.4^2 + 1/0.3^2)} = 0.576$$

$$\text{Weighted SE} = 0.24$$

$$\text{t - value} = 1.0/0.24 = 4.16$$

$$\text{p - value} = < 0.001$$

The weighted mean is equal to the unweighted mean. However, its SE is much smaller. It means that after adjustment for the prop scores a very significant difference is observed. Instead of subclassification, also linear regression with the propensity scores as covariate is a common way to deal with propensity scores. However, this is hard on a pocket calculator.

Propensity Score Matching

In a study of 200 patients each patient has his/her own propensity. We select for each patient in group 1 a patient from group 2 with the same propensity score. This procedure will end up sampling two new groups that are entirely symmetric on their subgroup variables, and can, thus, be simply analyzed as two groups in a randomized trial. In the given example two matched groups of 71 patients were left for comparison of the treatments. They can be analyzed for treatment differences using unpaired t-tests or Chi-square tests, without need to further account confounding anymore (Fig. 5.1).

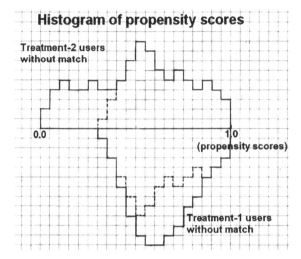

Fig. 5.1 The nearest neighbor watching method for matching patients with similar propensity scores. Each square represents one patient. In random order the first patient from group 1 is selected. Then, he/she is matched to the patient of group 2 with the nearest propensity score. We continue until there are no longer similar propensity scores. Group 1 is summarized above the x-axis, group 2 under it. The patients with dissimilar propensity score that can not be matched, are removed from the analysis

t-table. The t-values can be looked at as mean study results expressed in SEM-units. E.g., a mean study result expressed in units, mmol/l, g, etc., can also be expressed in SEM-units. This result is obtained if you divide the mean results by its own SEM. The upper row shows p-values = Areas under the curve (AUCs) of t-distributions. The second row gives two-sided p-values, it means that left and right end of the area under the curves of the Gaussian—like t-curves are added up. The left column gives degrees of freedom which are adjustments for the sample size. If it gets larger, then the corresponding Gaussian - like curves will get a bit narrower. In this manner the estimates become more precise and more in agreement with reality. The t-table is empirical, and has been constructed in the 30s of the past century with the help of simulation models and practical examples. It is till now the basis of modern statistics, and all modern software makes extensively use of it.

v	Q = 0.4	0.25	0.1	0.05	0.025	0.01	0.005	0.001
	2Q = 0.8	0.5	0.2	0.1	0.05	0.02	0.01	0.002
1	0.325	1.000	3.078	6.314	12.706	31.821	63.657	318.31
2	0.289	0.816	1.886	2.920	4.303	6.965	9.925	22.326
3	0.277	0.765	1.638	2.353	30182	4.547	5.841	10.213
4	0.171	0.741	1.533	2.132	2.776	3.747	4.604	7.173

(continued)

(continued)

5	0.267	0.727	1.476	2.015	2.571	3.365	4.032	5.893
6	0.265	0.718	1.440	1.943	20447	3.143	3.707	5.208
7	0.263	0.711	1.415	1.895	2.365	2.998	3.499	4.785
8	0.262	0.706	1.397	1.860	2.306	2.896	3.355	4.501
9	0.261	0.703	1.383	1.833	2.262	2.821	3.250	4.297
10	0.261	0.700	1.372	1.812	2.228	2.764	3.169	4.144
11	0.269	0.697	1.363	1.796	2.201	2.718	3.106	4.025
12	0.269	0.695	0.356	1.782	2.179	2.681	3.055	3.930
13	0.259	0.694	1.350	1.771	2.160	2.650	3.012	3.852
14	0.258	0.692	1.345	1.761	2.145	2.624	2.977	3.787
15	0.258	0.691	1.341	1.753	2.131	2.602	2.947	3.733
16	0.258	0.690	1.337	1.746	2.120	2.583	2.921	3.686
17	0.257	0.689	1.333	1.740	2.110	2.567	2.898	3.646
18	0.257	0.688	1.330	1.734	2.010	2.552	2.878	3.610
19	0.257	0.688	1.328	1.729	2.093	2.539	2.861	3.579
20	0.257	0.687	1.325	1.725	2.086	2.528	2.845	3.552
21	0.257	0.686	1.323	1.721	2.080	2.518	2.831	3.527
22	0.256	0.686	1.321	1.717	2.074	2.508	2.819	3.505
23	0.256	0.685	1.319	1.714	2.069	2.600	2.807	3.485
24	0.256	0.685	1.318	1.711	2.064	2.492	2.797	3.467
25	0.256	0.684	1.316	1.708	2.060	2.485	2.787	3.450
26	0.256	0.654	1.35	1.706	2.056	2.479	2.779	3.435
27	0.256	0.684	1.314	1.701	2.052	2.473	2.771	3.421
28	0.256	0.683	1.313	1.701	2.048	2.467	2.763	3.408
29	0.256	0.683	1.311	1.699	2.045	2.462	2.756	3.396
30	0.256	0.683	1.310	1.697	2.042	2.457	2.750	3.385
40	0.255	0.681	1.303	1.684	2.021	2.423	2.704	3.307
60	0.254	0.679	1.296	1.671	2.000	2.390	2.660	3.232
120	0.254	0.677	1.289	1.658	1.950	2.358	2.617	3.160
∞	0.253	0.674	1.282	1.645	1.960	2.326	2.576	3.090

Conclusion

Propensity scores are ideal for assessing confounding, particularly, if multiple confounders are in a study. Propensity score matching is used to make observational data look like randomized controlled trial data.

Chapter 6
Markov Modeling for Predicting Outside the Range of Observations

Regression models are only valid within the range of the x-values observed in the data. Markov modeling goes one step further, and aims at predicting outside the range of x-values. Like with Cox regression it assumes an exponential-pattern in the data which may be a strong assumption for complex human beings.

Example

In patients with diabetes mellitus type II, sulfonureas are highly efficacious, but they will, eventually, induce beta-cell failure. Beta-cell failure is defined as a fasting plasma glucose >7.0 mmol/l. The question is, does the severity of diabetes and/or the potency of the sulfonurea-compound influence the induction of beta-cell failure? This was studied in 500 patients with diabetes type II.

At time 0 year	0/500 patients	Had beta-cell failure
At time 1 year	50/500 patients (=10 %)	Had beta-cell failure.

As after 1 year 90 % had no beta-cell failure, it is appropriate according to the Markow model to extrapolate:

after 2 years 90 × 90 %   = 81 % no beta-cell failure.
after 3 years 90 × 90 × 90 % = 73 % no beta-cell failure.
after 6.58 years   = 50 % no beta-cell failure.

The calculation using logarithmic transformation is given in Chap. 2.

A second question was, does the severity of diabetes mellitus type II influence induction of beta-cell failure. A cut-off level for severity often applied is a fasting

T. J. Cleophas and A. H. Zwinderman, *Statistical Analysis of Clinical Data on a Pocket Calculator, Part 2*, SpringerBriefs in Statistics, DOI: 10.1007/978-94-007-4704-3_6,
© The Author(s) 2012

plasma glucose >10 mmol/l. According to the Markov modeling approach the question can be answered as follows:

250 patients had fasting plasma glucose <10 mmol/l at diagnosis (Group-1).
250 patients had fasting plasma glucose >10 mmol/l at diagnosis (Group-2).

If after 1 year sulfonureas (su) treatment, 10/250 of the patients from Group-1 had beta-cell failure, and 40/250 of the patients from Group-2, which is significantly different with an odds ratio of 0.22 (p < 0.01, see Chap. 2 for the calculation), then we can again extrapolate:

In Group-1 it takes 17 years before 50 % of the patients develop beta-cell failure.
In Group-2 it takes 4 years before 50 % of the patients develop beta-cell failure.

The next question is, does potency of su-compound influence induction of beta-cell failure?

250 patients started on amaryl (potent sulfonurea) at diagnosis (Group-A).
250 patients started on artosin (non-potent sulfonurea) at diagnosis (Group-B).

If after 1 year 25/250 of Group-A had beta-cell failure, and 25/250 of the Group-B, it is appropriate according to the Markov model to conclude that a non-potent does not prevent beta-cell failure.

Note

Markov modeling, although its use is very common in long-term observational studies, is highly speculative, because nature does not routinely follow mathematical models.

Conclusion

Regression models are only valid within the range of the x-values observed in the data. Markov modeling goes one step further, and aims at predicting outside the range of x-values.

Chapter 7
Uncertainty in the Evaluation of Diagnostic Tests

Sensitivity and specificity are measures of diagnostic accuracy of qualitative diagnostic tests, and are obtained from data samples. Just like averages they are estimates and come with certain amounts of uncertainty. The standards for reporting diagnostic accuracy (STARDS) working party recommends to include measures of uncertainty in any evaluation of a diagnostic test.

Estimating Uncertainty of Sensitivity and Specificity

For the calculation of the standard errors (SEs) of sensitivity , specificity and overall-validity we make use of the Gaussian curve assumption in the data.

		Definitive diagnosis (n)	
		Yes	No
Result diagnostic test	Yes	a	b
	No	c	d

Sensitivity = a/(a + c) = proportion true positives
Specificity = d/(b + d) = proportion true negatives
1-specificity = b/(b + d)
Proportion of patients with a definitive diagnosis = (a+c)/(a + b + c + d)
Overall validity = (a + d)/(a + b + c + d)
In order to make predictions from these estimates of validity their standard deviations/errors are required. The standard deviation/error (SD/SE) of a proportion can be calculated.

T. J. Cleophas and A. H. Zwinderman, *Statistical Analysis of Clinical Data on a Pocket Calculator, Part 2*, SpringerBriefs in Statistics, DOI: 10.1007/978-94-007-4704-3_7, © The Author(s) 2012

| SD = | $\sqrt{\ }$ p(1−p) where p = proportion. |
| SE = | $\sqrt{\ }$ [p(1−p)/n] where n = sample size |

where p equals a/(a + c) for the sensitivity. Using the above equations the standard error can be readily obtained.

SE $_{\text{specificity}}$ =	$\sqrt{\ }$ ac/(a + c)^3
SE $_{\text{specificity}}$ =	$\sqrt{\ }$ db/(d + b)^3
SE $_{\text{1-specificity}}$ =	$\sqrt{\ }$ db/(d + b)^3
SE $_{\text{proportion of patients with a definitive diagnosis}}$ =	$\sqrt{\ }$ (a + b)(c + d)/(a + b + c + d)^3

Example 1

Two hundred patients are evaluated the determine the sensitivity /specificity of B-type natriuretic peptide (BNP) for making a diagnosis of heart failure.

		Heart failure (n)	
		Yes	No
Result diagnostic test	Positive	70 (a)	35 (b)
	Negative	30 (c)	65 (d)

The sensitivity (a/(a + c)) and specificity (d/(b + d)) are calculated to be 0.70 and 0.65 respectively (70 and 65 %). In order for these estimates to be significantly larger than 50 % their 95 % confidence interval should not cross the 50 % boundary. The standard error are calculated using the above equations. For sensitivity the standard error is 0.0458, for specificity 0.0477. Under the assumption of Gaussian curve distributions in the data the 95 % confidence intervals of the sensitivity and specificity can be calculated according to:

95 % confidence interval of the sensitivity = 0.70 ± 1.96 × 0.0458
95 % confidence interval of the specificity = 0.65 ± 1.96 × 0.0477.

This means that the 95 % confidence interval of the sensitivity is between 61 and 79 %, for specificity it is between 56 and 74 %. These results do not cross the 50 % boundary and fall, thus, entirely within the boundary of validity. The diagnostic test can be accepted as being valid.

Example 2

Dimer tests have been widely used as screening tests for lung embolias.

		Lung embolia (n)	
		Yes	No
Dimer test	Positive	2 (a)	18 (b)
	Negative	1 (c)	182 (d)

The sensitivity (a/(a + c)) and specificity (d/(b + d)) are calculated to be 0.666 and 0.911 respectively (67 and 91%). In order for these estimates to be significantly larger than 50 % the 95 % confidence interval of them should again not cross the 50 % boundary.

The standard error , as calculated according to the above equations, are for sensitivity 0.272, for specificity 0.040. Under the assumption of Gaussian curve distributions the 95 % confidence intervals of the sensitivity and specificity are calculated according to:

95 % confidence interval of the sensitivity $= 0.67 \pm 1.96 \times 0.272$
95 % confidence interval of the specificity $= 0.91 \pm 1.96 \times 0.040$.

The 95 % confidence interval of the sensitivity is between 0.14 and 1.20 (14 and 120 %). The 95 % confidence interval of the specificity can be similarly calculated, and is between 0.87 and 0.95 (87 and 95 %). The interval for the sensitivity is very wide and does not at all fall within the boundaries of 0.5–1.0 (50–100 %). Validity of this test is, therefore, not really demonstrated. The appropriate conclusion of this evaluation should be: based on this evaluation the diagnostic cannot be accepted as being valid in spite of a sensitivity and specificity of respectively 67 and 91 %.

Conclusion

Sensitivity and specificity are estimates of accurancy of diagnostic tests. They come with certain amounts of uncertainty. Methods for the purpose are explained.

Chapter 8
Robust Tests for Imperfect Data

Robust tests are tests that can handle the inclusion of some outliers into a data file without largely changing the overall test results. Frailty score-improvements after physiotherapy of 33 patients are measured in a study (second column of underneath data).

Patient	Score-improvement	Deviation from median	Trimmed data	Winsorized data
1	−8.00	11		−1.00
2	−8.00	11		−1.00
3	−8.00	7		−1.00
4	−4.00	7		−1.00
5	−4.00	7		−1.00
6	−4.00	7		−1.00
7	−4.00	7		−1.00
8	−1.00	4	-1.00	−1.00
9	0.00	3	0.00	0.00
10	0.00	3	0.00	0.00
11	0.00	3	0.00	0.00
12	1.00	2	1.00	1.00
13	1.00	2	1.00	1.00
14	2.00	1	2.00	2.00
15	2.00	1	2.00	2.00
16	2.00	1	2.00	2.00
17	3.00	Median	3.00	3.00
18	3.00	0	3.00	3.00
19	3.00	0	3.00	3.00
20	3.00	0	3.00	3.00
21	4.00	1	4.00	4.00
22	4.00	1	4.00	4.00
23	4.00	1	4.00	4.00

(continued)

T. J. Cleophas and A. H. Zwinderman, *Statistical Analysis of Clinical Data on a Pocket Calculator, Part 2*, SpringerBriefs in Statistics, DOI: 10.1007/978-94-007-4704-3_8, © The Author(s) 2012

(continued)

Patient	Score-improvement	Deviation from median	Trimmed data	Winsorized data
24	4.00	1	4.00	4.00
25	5.00	2	5.00	5.00
26	5.00	2	5.00	5.00
27	5.00	2		5.00
28	5.00	2		5.00
29	6.00	3		5.00
30	6.00	3		5.00
31	6.00	3		5.00
32	7.00	4		5.00
33	8.00	5		5.00

Table 8.1 Descriptives of the data

Mean	1.455
Standard deviation	4.409
Standard error	0.768
Mean after replacing outcome 1st patient with 0.00	1.697
Mean after replacing outcome first 3 patients with 0.00	2.182
Median	3.000
MAD	2.500
Mean of the Winsorized data	1.364
Standard deviation of the Winsorized data	3.880

MAD = median absolute deviation = the median value of the sorted deviations from the median of a data file

The data suggest the presence of some central tendency: the values 3.00 and 5.00 are observed more frequently than the rest. However, the one sample t-test (see part 1 of this title page 5) shows a mean difference from zero of 1.45 scores with a p-value of 0.067. Thus, not statistically significant from zero.

T-test for Medians and Median Absolute Deviations (MADs)

If the mean does not accurately reflect the central tendency of the data e.g., in case of outliers (highly unusual values), then the median (value in the middle) or the mode (value most frequently observed) may be a better alternative to summarizing the data and making predictions from them. The above example is used.

Median = 3.00

The above example shows in the third column the deviations from the median, and Table 8.1 gives the median of the deviations from median (MAD = median absolute deviation).

MAD = 2.50

If we assume, that the data, though imperfect, are from a normal distribution, then the standard deviation of this normal distribution can be approximated from the equation

standard deviation$_{median}$ = 1.426 × MAD = 3.565

standard error$_{median}$ = 3.565/$\sqrt{}$ n = 3.565/$\sqrt{}$ 33 = 0.6206

A t-test (t-table in Chap. 5) is subsequently performed, and produces a very significant effect: physiotherapy is really helpful.

t = median/standard error$_{median}$ = 3.00/0.6206 = 4.834

p-value < 0.0001

T-test for Winsorized Variances

The terminology comes from Winsor's principle: all observed distributions are Gaussian in the middle. First, we have to trim the data, e.g., by 20 % on either side (see data file, fourth column). Then, we have to fill up their trimmed values with Winsorized scores, which are the smallest and largest untrimmed scores (data file, fifth column). The mean is then calculated as well as the standard deviation and standard error, and a t-test (t-table in Chap. 5) is performed for null hypothesis testing.

Winsorized mean = 1.364
Winsorized standard deviation = 3.880
Winsorized standard error = 3.880/$\sqrt{n}$
                                  = 3.880/$\sqrt{}$ 33
                                  = 0.675
t-test
t = Winsorized mean/Winsorized standard error
t = 2.021
p-value = 0.0433

Mood's Test (One Sample Wilcoxon's Test)

This test is sometimes called the one sample Wilcoxon's test. Table 8.2 shows how it works. Paired averages [(vertical value + horizontal value)/2] are calculated. If the data are equally distributed around an average of 0, then we will have half of the average being positive, half negative.

We observe

1122 paired averages,
1122/2 = 561 should be positive,
349 positive paired averages are found.
Chi-square test (see Chi-square table in Chap. 4)

Table 8.2 Partial presentation of paired averages of the data from the above example

	−8.00	−8.00	−8.00	−4.00	−4.00	−4.00	−1.00	0.00	0.00	0.00	1.00 ....
−8.00	−8.00	−8.00	−6.00	−6.00	−6.00	−4.50	−4.00	−4.00	−4.00	−3.50
−8.00		−8.00	−6.00	−6.00	−6.00	−4.50	−4.00	−4.00	−4.00	−3.50
−8.00			−6.00	−6.00	−6.00	−4.50	−4.00	−4.00	−4.00	−3.50
−4.00				−4.00	−4.00	−2.50	−2.00	−2.00	−2.00	−1.50
−4.00					−4.00	−2.50	−2.00	−2.00	−2.00	−1.50
−4.00						−2.50	−2.00	−2.00	−2.00	−1.50
−1.00							−0.50	−0.50	−0.50	0.00
0.00								0.00	0.00	0.50
0.00									0.00	0.50
0.00										0.50
1.00										
....
....

Chi-square value = (Observed−expected numbers)^2/Expected numbers
Chi-square value = $(349−561)^2/349 = 128.729$
p < 0.0001 with 1 degree of freedom

The above three robust tests produced p-values of <0.0001, 0.043, and <0.0001, while the one sample t-test was not statistically significant. Robust tests are wonderful for imperfect data, because they often produce significant results, when standard tests don't.

Conclusion

Robust tests are tests that can handle the inclusion of some outliers into a data file without largely changing the overall test results. The tests are explained.

Chapter 9
Non-Linear Modeling on a Pocket Calculator

Non-linear relationships in clinical research are often linear after logarithmic transformations. Odds ratios, log likelihood ratios, Markov models and many regression models are models that make use of it. An example with real data is given. We have to add that logarithmic transformation is not always successful, and that alternative methods are available like Box Cox transformation, and computationally intensive methods like spline and Loess modeling (see Chap. 24. In: Statistics Applied to Clinical Studies, Springer New York, 5th edition, 2012, and the Chap. 14 of "SPSS for Starters", Part 2, Springer New York, 2012, both from the same authors). However, these methods generally require statistical software and can not be executed on a pocket calculator.

Example

Figure 9.1 shows the survivals of 240 patients with small cell carcinomas, and Fig. 9.2 shows the natural logarithms of these survivals. From Fig. 9.2 it can be observed that logarithmic transformation of the numbers of patients alive readily produces a close to linear pattern. The equation of the regression line of Fig. 9.2 $y = a + bx$ with a = intercept and b = regression coefficient can be calculated on a pocket calculator (see appendix).

Appendix

Linear Regression ($y = a + bx$, r = Correlation Coefficient)

Some pocket calculators offer linear regression. An example is given.

T. J. Cleophas and A. H. Zwinderman, *Statistical Analysis of Clinical Data on a Pocket Calculator, Part 2*, SpringerBriefs in Statistics, DOI: 10.1007/978-94-007-4704-3_9, © The Author(s) 2012

Fig. 9.1 Survivals of 240 random patients with small cell carcinomas

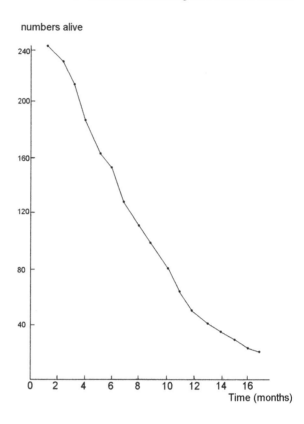

x-values [temp (°C)]	y-values [atmospheric pressure (hpa)]
10	1003
15	1005
20	1010
25	1011
30	1014

Electronic Calculator, Kenko KK-82MS-5

Press: on....mode....3....1....10..., ...1003....M+....15....,   1005....
M+.....etc....M+....shift....s-var...▶...▶....1....a is given...
     shift....s-var...▶...▶....2....b is given.... shift....s-var...▶...▶....3....r is given...

Fig. 9.2 The logarithmic transformation of the numbers of patients from Fig. 9.1 produces a close to linear pattern

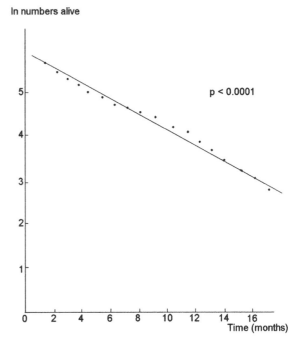

Interpretation of a, b and r.: a is the intercept of the best fit regression line with equation y = a + bx; b is the regression coefficient, otherwise called direction coefficient of the regression line; r is Pearson's correlation coefficient, it runs from -1 to $+1$, 0 means no relationships between x and y, -1 and $+1$ mean a very strong negative and positive relationship respectively.

Conclusion

Non-linear relationships in clinical research are often linear after logarithmic transformation. An example is given.

Chapter 10
Fuzzy Modeling for Imprecise and Incomplete Data

Fuzzy modeling is a methodology that works with partial truths: it can answer questions to which the answers are "yes" and "no" at different times or partly "yes" and "no" at the same time. It can be used to match any type of data, particularly incomplete and imprecise data, and it is able to improve precision of such data. It can be applied with any type of statistical distribution and it is, particularly, suitable for uncommon and unexpected non linear relationships.

Fuzzy Terms

Universal space.

Defined range of imput values, defined range of output values.

Fuzzy memberships.

The universal spaces are divided into equally sized parts called membership functions.

Linguistic membership names.

Each fuzzy membership is given a name, otherwise called linguistic term.

Triangular fuzzy sets.

A common way of drawing the membership function with on the x-axis the imput values, on the y-axis the membership grade for each imput value.

T. J. Cleophas and A. H. Zwinderman, *Statistical Analysis of Clinical Data on a Pocket Calculator, Part 2*, SpringerBriefs in Statistics, DOI: 10.1007/978-94-007-4704-3_10, © The Author(s) 2012

Table 10.1 Quantal pharmacodynamic effects of different induction dosages of thiopental on numbers of responding subjects

Imput values	Output values	Fuzzy-modeled output
Induction dosage of thiopental (mg/kg)	Numbers of responders (n)	Numbers of thiopental responders (n)
1	4	4
1.5	5	6
2	6	8
2.5	9	10
3	12	12
3.5	17	14
4	17	16
4.5	12	14
5	9	12

Fuzzy plots.

Graphs summarizing the fuzzy memberships of (for example) the imput values (Fig. 10.2 upper graph).

Linguistic rules.

The relationships between the fuzzy memberships of the imput data and those of the output data (the method of calculation is shown in the underneath examples).

Example

The effects of different induction dosages of thiopental on numbers of responding subjects are in Table 10.1, left two columns. The right column gives the fuzzy-modeled output. Figure 10.1 shows that the un-modeled curve (upper curve) fits the data less well than does the modeled (lower curve).

We fuzzy-model the imput and output relationships (Fig. 10.2).

First of all, we create linguistic rules for the imput and output data.

For that purpose we divide the universal space of the imput variable into fuzzy memberships with linguistic membership names:

imput-*zero*, -*small*, -*medium*, -*big*, -*superbig*.

Then we do the same for the output variable:

output-*zero*, -*small*, -*medium*, -*big*.

Subsequently, we create linguistic rules.

Figure 10.2 shows that imput-*zero* consists of the values 1 and 1.5.

The value 1 (100 % membership) has 4 as outcome value (100 % membership of output-*zero*).

Example 37

Fig. 10.1 Pharmacodynamic relationship between induction dose of thiopental (x-axis, mg/kg) and number of responders (y-axis). The un-modeled curve (*upper curve*) fits the data less well than does the modeled (*lower curve*)

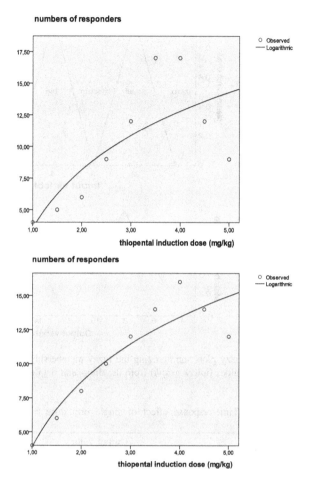

The value 1.5 (50 % membership) has 5 as outcome value (75 % membership of output-*zero*, 25 % of output-*small*).

The imput-*zero* produces 100 % × 100 % + 50 % × 75 % = 137.5 % membership to output-*zero*, and 50 % × 25 % = 12.5 % membership to output-*small*, and so, output-*zero* is the most important output contributor here, and we forget about the small contribution of output-*small*.

Imput-*small* is more complex, it consists of the values 1.5, and 2.0, and 2.5.

The value 1.5 (50 % membership) has 5 as outcome value (75 % membership of output-*zero*, 25 % membership of output-*small*).

The value 2.0 (100 % membership) has 6 as outcome value (50 % membership of outcome-*zero*, and 50 % membership of output-*small*).

The value 2.5 (50 % membership) has 9 as outcome value (75 % membership of output-*small* and 25 % of output-*medium*).

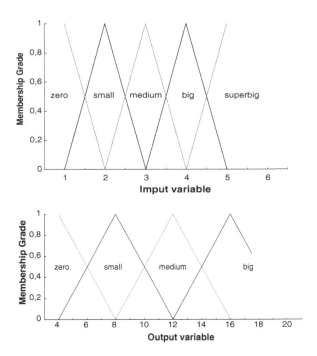

Fig. 10.2 Fuzzy plots summarizing the fuzzy memberships of the imput values (*upper graph*) and output values (*lower graph*) from the thiopental data (Table 10.1 and Fig. 10.1)

Table 10.2 Time-response effect of single oral dose of 120 mg propranolol on peripheral arterial flow

Imput values	Output values	Fuzzy-modeled output
Hours after oral Administration of 120 mg propranolol	Peripheral arterial flow (ml/100 ml tissue/min)	Peripheral arterial flow (ml/100 ml tissue/min)
1	20	20
2	12	14
3	9	8
4	6	6
5	5	4
6	4	4
7	5	4
8	6	6
9	9	8
10	12	14
11	20	20

The imput-*small* produces $50\% \times 75\% + 100\% \times 50\% = 87.5\%$ membership to output-*zero*, $50\% \times 25\% + 100\% \times 50\% + 50\% \times 75\% = 100\%$ membership to output-*small*, and $50\% \times 25\% = 12.5\%$ membership to

Example   39

Fig. 10.3 Pharmacodynamic relationship between the time after oral administration of 120 mg of propranolol (x-axis, hours) and absolute change in fore arm flow (y-axis, ml/100 ml tissue/min). The un-modeled curve (*upper curve*) fits the data slightly less well than does the modeled (*lower curve*)

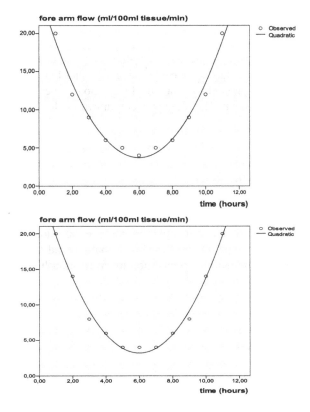

output-*medium*. And so, the output-*small* is the most important contributor here, and we forget about the other two.

For the other imput memberships similar linguistic rules are determined:

Imput-*medium* → output-*medium*
Imput-*big* → output-*big*
Imput-*superbig* → output-*medium*

We are, particularly interested in the modeling capacity of fuzzy logic in order to improve the precision of pharmacodynamic modeling.

The modeled output value of imput value 1 is found as follows.

Value 1 is 100 % member of imput-*zero*, meaning that according to the above linguistic rules it is also associated with a 100 % membership of output-*zero* corresponding with a value of 4.

Value 1.5 is 50 % member of imput-*zero* and 50 % imput-*small*. This means it is 50 % associated with the output-*zero* and -*small* corresponding with values of 50 % × (4 + 8) = 6.

For all of the imput values modeled output values can be found in this way. Table 10.1 right column shows the results.

Example for Exercise

In the next example the fuzzy-modeled output has been given. Try and fuzzy-model the data for yourself (Table 10.2 and Fig. 10.3).

The figures show that the fuzzy models better fit the data than do the un-modeled data. The figures were drawn with SPSS module regression (curve estimation).

Conclusion

Fuzzy modeling can be used to match any type of data, particularly incomplete and imprecise data, and it is able to improve precision of such data. It can be applied with any type of statistical distribution and it is, particularly, suitable for uncommon and unexpected non linear relationships.

Chapter 11
Goodness of Fit Tests for Normal and Cumulatively Normal Data

Goodness of fit with the normal distribution or cumulatively normal distribution of a data file is an important requirement for a normal or rank test to be sensitive for testing the data. Data files that lack goodness of fit can be analyzed using distribution free methods, like Monte Carlo modeling and neural network modeling (SPSS for Starters, Part 2 from the same authors, Springer New York, 2012).

Chi-Square Goodness of Fit Test

In random populations body-weights follow a normal distribution. Is this also true for the body-weights of a group of patients treated with a weight reducing compound?

Individual weight (kgs)

85	57	60	81	89	63	52	65	77	64
89	86	90	60	57	61	95	78	66	92
50	56	95	60	82	55	61	81	61	53
63	75	50	98	63	77	50	62	79	69
76	66	97	67	54	93	70	80	67	73

The area under the curve (AUC) of a normal distribution curve is divided into 5 equiprobable intervals of 20 % each, we expect approximately 10 patients per interval. From the data a mean and standard deviation (sd) of 71 and 15 kg are calculated. Figure 11.1 shows that the standardized cut-off results (z-values) for the five intervals are -0.84, -0.025, 0.25 and 0.84. The real cut-off results are calculated according to

$$z = \text{standardized result} = \frac{\text{unstandardized result} - \text{mean result}}{sd}$$

T. J. Cleophas and A. H. Zwinderman, *Statistical Analysis of Clinical Data on a Pocket Calculator, Part 2*, SpringerBriefs in Statistics, DOI: 10.1007/978-94-007-4704-3_11,

Fig. 11.1 The standardized cut-off results (z-value) for the five intervals with an AUC of 20 % are −0.84, −0.25, 0.25, and 0.84 (AUC = area under the curve)

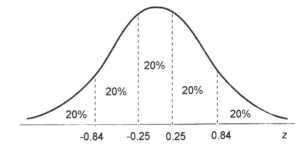

and are given below (pts = patients).

$$\text{Intervals(kgs)} \quad -\infty \quad 58.40 \quad 67.25 \quad 74.25 \quad 83.60 \quad \infty$$

| As they are equiprobable, we expect per interval: | 10 pts I 10 pts I 10 pts I 10 pts I 10pts |
| We do, however, observe the following numbers: | 10 pts I 16 pts I 3 pts I 10 pts I 11pts |

The Chi-square value is calculated according to

$$\sum \frac{(\text{observed number} - \text{expected number})^2}{\text{expected number}} = 8.6$$

This Chi-square value means that for the given degrees of freedom of $5-1 = 4$ (there are five different intervals) the null-hypothesis of no-difference-between-observed-and-expected can not be rejected (Chi-square table, Chap. 4). However, our p-value is <0.10, and, so, there is a trend of a difference. The data may not be entirely normal, as expected. This may be due to lack of randomness.

Kolmogorov–Smirnov Goodness of Fit Test

In random populations plasma cholesterol levels follow a normal distribution. Is this also true for the plasma cholesterol levels of the underneath patients treated with a cholesterol reducing compound?

Cholesterol (mmol/l)	<4.01	4.01–5.87	5.87–7.73	7.73–9.59	>9.59
Numbers of pts	13	158	437	122	20

Fig. 11.2 The standardized cut-off results (z-values) for the five intervals are calculated to be −2.25, −0.75, 0.75, and 2.25. Corresponding AUCs are given in the graph (AUC = area under the curve)

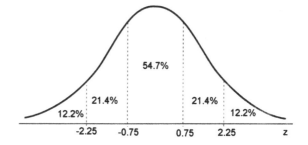

The cut-off results for the five intervals must be standardized to find the expected normal distribution for these data according to

$$z = \text{standardized cut} - \text{off result} = \frac{\text{unstandardized result - mean result}}{\text{sd.}}$$

With a calculated mean (sd) of 6.80 (1.24) we find −2.25, −0.75, 0.75 and 2.25. Figure 11.2 gives the distribution graph plus AUCs. With 750 cholesterol-values in total the expected frequencies of cholesterol-values in the subsequent intervals are

$$12.2 \times 750 = 9.2$$
$$21.4 \times 750 = 160.8$$
$$54.7 \times 750 = 410.1$$
$$21.4 \times 750 = 160.8$$
$$12.2 \times 750 = 9.2$$

The observed and expected frequencies are, then, listed cumulatively (cumul = cumulative):

Frequency observed	Cumul	Relative (cumul/750)	Expected	Cumul	Relative (cumul/750)	Cumul observed− expected
13	13	0.0173	9.2	9.1	0.0122	0.0051
158	171	0.2280	0.2280	170.0	0.2266	0.0014
437	608	0.8107	0.8107	580.1	0.7734	0.0373
122	730	0.9733	0.9733	740.9	0.9878	0.0145
20	750	1.000	1.000	750	1.000	0.00000

According to the Kolmogorov–Smirnov table (Table 11.1) the largest cumulative difference between observed and expected should be smaller than $1.36/\sqrt{n} = 1.36/\sqrt{750} = 0.0497$, while we find 0.0373. This means that these data are well normally distributed. We should add that a positive Kolmogorov–Smirnov test not only indicates that normal testing is not warranted, but also that rank

Table 11.1 Critical values of the Kolmogorov–Smirnov goodness of fit test

Samplesize(n)	Level of statistical significance for maximum difference between cumulative observed and expected frequency				
n	0.20	0.15	0.10	0.05	0.01
1	0.900	0.925	0.950	0.975	0.995
2	0.684	0.726	0.776	0.824	0.929
3	0.565	0.597	0.642	0.708	0.828
4	0.494	0.525	0.564	0.624	0.733
5	0.446	0.474	0.470	0.565	0.669
6	0.410	0.436	0.438	0.521	0.618
7	0.381	0.405	0.411	0.486	0.577
8	0.358	0.381	0.388	0.457	0.543
9	0.339	0.360	0.368	0.432	0.514
10	0.322	0.342	0.352	0.410	0.490
11	0.307	0.326	0.338	0.391	0.468
12	0.295	0.313	0.325	0.375	0.450
13	0.284	0.302	0.314	0.361	0.463
14	0.274	0.292	0.304	0.349	0.418
15	0.266	0.283	0.295	0.338	0.404
16	0.258	0.274	0.286	0.328	0392
17	0.250	0.266	0.278	0.318	0.381
18	0.244	0.259	0.272	0.309	0.371
19	0.237	0.252	0.264	0.301	0.363
20	0.231	0.246	0.24	0.294	0.356
25	0.21	0.22	0.22	0.27	0.32
30	0.19	0.20	0.21	0.24	0.29
35	0.18	0.19	1.21	0.23	0.27
Over 35	$1.07\sqrt{n}$	$1.14\sqrt{n}$	$1.22\sqrt{n}$	$1.36\sqrt{n}$	$1.63\sqrt{n}$

testing like non-parametric testing (see complementary book from the same authors, SPSS for Starters, Part 1, Chaps. 3 and 4) is not to be recommended, as Kolmogorow–Smirnov tests are based on a normal distribution of the data after cumulative ranking of the data.

Conclusion

Goodness of fit with the normal distribution or cumulatively normal distribution is an important requirement for a normal or rank test to be sensitive for testing the data. Data files that lack goodness of fit can be analyzed using distribution free methods, like Monte Carlo modeling and neural network modeling (SPSS for Starters. Part 2 from the same authors. Springer New York. 2012).

Chapter 12
Bhattacharya Modeling for Unmasking Hidden Gaussian Curves

Bhattacharya modeling can be used for unmasking Gaussian curves in the data. It is applied for determining normal values of diagnostic tests and their confidence intervals, and for searching subsets in the data.

Example

Figure 12.1 gives an example of the frequency distributions of vascular lab scores of a population of 787 patients at risk of peripheral vascular disease. The pattern of the histogram is suggestive of certain subsets in this population. The Table 12.1 left two columns give the scores and frequencies. The frequencies are log (logarithmic) transformed (third column) (see also Chap. 2), and, then, the differences between two subsequent log transformed scores are calculated (fourth column).

Figure 12.2 show the plot of the scores against the delta log terms. Three straight lines are identified. The equations of these lines can be calculated (using linear regression, see appendix in Chap. 9) or extrapolated from the Fig. 12.2.

1. $y = 0.944 - 0.078\, x$
2. $y = 0.692 - 0.026\, x$
3. $y = 2.166 - 0.048\, x$

The characteristics of the corresponding Gaussian curves can be calculated as follows.

1. mean $= -0.944/-0.078 = 12.10$, Standard deviation $= 1/0.078 = 12.82$
2. mean $= -0.692/-0.026 = 26.62$, Standard deviation $= 1/0.026 = 38.46$
3. mean $= -2.166/-0.048 = 45.13$, Standard deviation $= 1/0.048 = 20.83$.

T. J. Cleophas and A. H. Zwinderman, *Statistical Analysis of Clinical Data on a Pocket Calculator, Part 2*, SpringerBriefs in Statistics, DOI: 10.1007/978-94-007-4704-3_12,

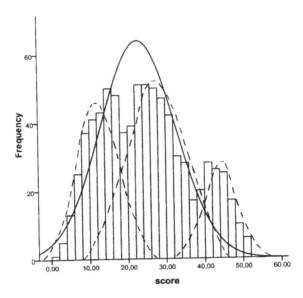

Fig. 12.1 The frequency distributions of vascular lab score is of 787 patients at risk of peripheral vascular disease. The continuous Gaussian curve is calculated from the mean ±standard deviation, the interrupted Gaussian curves from Bhattacharya modeling

Table 12.1 The frequency distribution of the vascular lab scores of 787 patients at risk of peripheral vascular disease (the data of Fig. 4). The log and delta log terms are respectively log transformations of the frequencies and differences between two subsequent log transformations

Score	Frequency	log	Delta log
2	1	0.000	0.000
4	5	0.699	0.699
6	13	1.114	0.415
8	25	1.398	0.284
10	37	1.568	0.170
12	41	1.613	0.045
14	43	1.633	0.020
16	50	1.699	−0.018
18	48	1.681	−0.111
20	37	1.570	0.021
22	39	1.591	0.117
24	51	1.708	0.000
26	51	1.708	−0.009
28	50	1.699	−0.027
30	47	1.672	−0.049
32	42	1.623	−0.146
34	30	1.477	−0.176
36	28	1.447	−0.030
38	16	1.204	−0.243

(continued)

Example 47

Table 12.1 (continued)

Score	Frequency	log	Delta log
40	20	1.301	0.097
42	28	1.447	0.146
44	26	1.415	−0.032
46	25	1.398	−0.017
48	17	1.230	−0.168
50	10	1.000	−0.230
52	6	0.778	−0.222

Fig. 12.2 The scores from Fig. 12.1 plotted against the delta log terms as calculated from the frequencies from Fig. 12.1

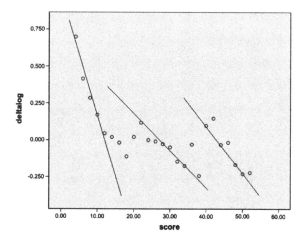

In Fig. 12.1 the above three Gaussian curves as given are drawn as interrupted curves.

We conclude that Bhattacharya modeling enables to identify Gaussian subsets in the data. It can also be applied to produce a better Gaussian fit to a data file than the usual mean and standard deviation does (Chap. 59. In: Statistics Applied to Clinical Studies, Springer New York, 5th edition, 2012, from the same authors).

Conclusion

Bhattacharya modeling can be used for unmasking Gaussian curves in the data. It is applied for determining normal values of diagnostic tests and their confidence intervals, and for searching subsets in the data. The methodology is explained.

.

Chapter 13
Item Response Modeling Instead of Classical Linear Analysis of Questionnaires

Item response modeling is used for analyzing psychometric data, quality of life data, and can even be used analyzing diagnostic tests. It provides better precision than does the classical linear analysis. An example with simulated data is given.

Example

One of the estimators of quality of life (QOL) is "feeling happy". Five yes/no questions indicate increasing levels of daily happiness: (1) morning, (2) afternoon, (3) night, (4) weekend, (5) daily. Usually, with five yes/no questions in a domain the individual result is given in the form of a score, here, e.g., a score from 0 to 5 dependent on the number of positive answers given per person. However, with many questionnaires different questions represent different levels of difficulty or different levels of benefit etc. This can be included in the analysis using item response modeling. Table 13.1 shows how 5 questions can be used to produce 32 different answer patterns. The Fig. 13.1 shows a histogram of the answer patterns

T. J. Cleophas and A. H. Zwinderman, *Statistical Analysis of Clinical Data on a Pocket Calculator, Part 2*, SpringerBriefs in Statistics, DOI: 10.1007/978-94-007-4704-3_13,

Table 13.1 A summary of a 5-item quality of life data of 1,000 anginal patients

No. response pattern	Response pattern (1 = yes, 2 = no) to items 1–5	Observed frequencies
1.	11111	0
2.	11112	0
3.	11121	0
4.	11122	1
5.	11211	2
6.	11212	3
7.	11221	5
8.	11222	8
9.	12111	12
10.	12112	15
11.	12121	18
12.	12122	19
13.	12211	20
14.	12212	21
15.	12221	21
16.	12222	21
17.	21111	20
18.	21112	19
19.	21121	18
20.	21122	15
21.	21211	12
22.	21212	9
23.	21221	5
24.	21222	3
25.	22111	4
26.	22112	0
27.	22121	0
28.	22122	0
29.	22211	0
30.	22212	0
31.	22221	0
32.	22222	0
		271

with the type of pattern on the x-axis and "how often" on the y-axis. A Gaussian like distribution frequency is observed. A score around 15 is observed most frequently, and can be interpreted as the mean score of the study. Low scores indicate little QOL. High scores indicate high QOL. The areas under the curve (AUCs) of the histogram is given on the next page. The larger the AUCs, which run from 0.004 to 1.000 (0.4 to 100 %), the better the QOL.

Example   51

Fig. 13.1 Histogram of the answer patterns with the type of pattern on the x-axis and "how often"on the y-axis

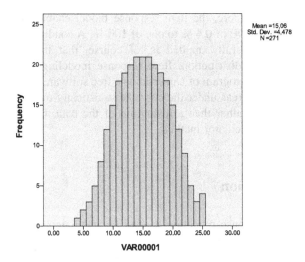

Response pattern	AUC (area under the curve)
4	1/271 = 0.004 (=4 %)
5	3 = 0.011
6	6 = 0.022
7	11 = 0.041
8	19 = 0.070
9	31 = 0.114
10	46 = 0.170
11	64 = 0.236
12	83 = 0.306
13	103 = 0.380
14	124 = 0.458
15	145 = 0.535
16	166 = 0.613
17	186 = 0.686
18	205 = 0.756
19	223 = 0.823
20	238 = 0.878
21	250 = 0.923
22	259 = 0.956
23	264 = 0.974
24	267 = 0.985
25	271 = 1.000 (=100 %)

Item response models are more sensitive than classical linear methods for making predictions from psychological/QOL questionnaires, and diagnostic tests. The above example shows that instead of a 6 point score running from 0 to 5 in the classical score, the item response model enabled to provide 32 scores, running from a QOL of 0.4 % to one of 100 %. A condition for item response modeling to be successfully applied is, of course, that the data should somewhat fit the Gaussian distribution. Item response modeling is not in SPSS, but the LTA-2 software program of Uebersax is a free software program for the purpose. It works with the areas under the curve of statistically modeled best fit Gaussian curves of the data rather than a histogram of the data, but, otherwise, it is similar to the pocket calculator method.

Conclusion

Item response modeling is used for analyzing psychometric data, quality of life data, and can even be used analyzing diagnostic tests. It provides better precision than does the classical linear analysis. The methodology is explained.

Chapter 14
Superiority Testing Instead of Null Hypothesis Testing

For this chapter some knowledge of power equations is required. This is given in Chap. 7 of the first part of this title. Superiority testing of a study means testing whether the study meets its a priori defined expected power. Many therapeutic studies may be able to reject their null hypotheses, and, are, thus, statistically significant, but they do not meet their expected power. Although p-values are widely reported, power is rarely given in the report. This may be a problem in practice, since lack of power indicates that the treatments are less efficacious than expected. Superiority testing assesses whether the eventual power of a study is in agreement with the power as stated in the sample size calculation of the study.

Example

The expected power of a study of a 10 patient crossover study is 90 %. The results of the study are given underneath:
observation 1:
6.0, 7.1, 8.1, 7.5, 6.4, 7.9, 6.8, 6.6, 7.3, 5.6
observation 2:
5.1, 8.0, 3.8, 4.4, 5.2, 5.4, 4.3, 6.0, 3.7, 6.2
Individual differences
0.9, −0.9, 4.3, 3.1, 1.2, 2.5, 2.5, 0.6, 3.8, −0.6
Is there a significant difference between the observation 1 and 2, and which level of significance is correct?

Mean difference $= 1.59$
SD of mean difference $= 1.789$
$SE = SD/\sqrt{10} = 0.566$
$t = 1.59/0.566 = 2.809$
$10-1 = 9$ degrees of freedom (10 patients and 1 group of patients).

T. J. Cleophas and A. H. Zwinderman, *Statistical Analysis of Clinical Data on a Pocket Calculator, Part 2*, SpringerBriefs in Statistics, DOI: 10.1007/978-94-007-4704-3_14,
© The Author(s) 2012

Look at the t-table (Chap. 5) to find the p-value. The ninth row shows that our t-value is between 2.262 and 2.821, this would mean a p-value between 0.05 and 0.02. There is, thus, a significant difference between observation 1 and 2. However, is the expected power obtained or is this study underpowered. The t-table is helpful to calculate the t-value required for a power of 90 %: it mean a beta-value (type II error value) of 10 % (= 0.1). Look at the upper row of the t-table.

If beta = 0.1, then

z_{beta} for 9 degrees of freedom = 1.383 (see note at the bottom).

The t-value required for a power of 90 %

= $1.383 + t^1$, where t^1 is the 0.05.

= 1.383 + 2.262

= 3.645.

The required t-value is much larger than the obtained t-value of 2.809, and, so, the study does not meet its expected power. The treatment is less efficacious than expected.

If the investigators had required a power of 60 %, then the superiority testing would be as follows.

beta = 0.40

z = 0.261

The t-value required for a power of 60 %

= $0.261 + t^1$, where t^1 is the 0.05.

= 0.261 + 2.262

= 2.523.

This t-value is smaller than the obtained t-value of 2.809, and, so, the study would have met an expected power of 60 %.

Note

The terms z-value and t-values are often used interchangeably, but strictly the z-value is the test statistic of the z-test, and the t-value is the test statistic of the t-test. The bottom row of the t-table is equal to the z-table.

Conclusion

Superiority testing of a study means testing whether the study meets its a priori defined expected power. Many therapeutic studies may be able to reject their null hypotheses, and, are, thus, statistically significant, but they do not meet their expected power. Although p-values are widely reported, power is rarely so. This may be a problem in practice, since lack of power indicates that the treatments are less efficacious than expected. Superiority testing assesses whether the eventual power of a study is in agreement with the power as stated in the sample size calculation prior to the study.

Chapter 15
Variability Analysis With the Bartlett's Test

In some clinical studies, the spread of the data may be more relevant than the average of the data. E.g., when we assess how a drug reaches various organs, variability of drug concentrations is important, as in some cases too little and in other cases dangerously high levels get through. Also, variabilities in drug response may be important. For example, the spread of glucose levels of a slow-release-insulin is important. In part 1 of this title, Chap. 16, the Chi-square test for one sample and the F-test for two samples have been explained. In this chapter we will explain the Bartlett's test which is suitable for comparing two samples, but can also be used for comparing multiple samples.

Example (Bartlett's Test)

$$\chi^2 = (n_1 + n_2 + n_3 - 3) \ln s^2 - [(n_1 - 1) \ln s_1^2 + (n_2 - 1) \ln s_2^2 + (n_3 - 1) \ln s_3^2]$$
where n_1 = size sample 1
s_1^2 = variance sample 1
s^2 = pooled variance = $\dfrac{(n_1 - 1)s_1^2 + (n_2 - 1)s_2^2 + (n_3 - 1)s_3^2}{n_1 + n_2 + n_3 - 3}$
$\ln$ = natural logarithm

As an example, blood glucose variabilities are assessed in a parallel-group study of three insulin treatment regimens. For that purpose three different groups of patients are treated with different insulin regimens. Variabilities of blood glucose levels are estimated by group-variances ($\ln$ = natural logarithm, see also Chap. 2):

	Group size (n)	Variance [$(mmol/l)^2$]
Group 1	100	8.0
Group 2	100	14.0
Group 3	100	18.0

T. J. Cleophas and A. H. Zwinderman, *Statistical Analysis of Clinical Data on a Pocket Calculator, Part 2*, SpringerBriefs in Statistics, DOI: 10.1007/978-94-007-4704-3_15, © The Author(s) 2012

$$\text{Pooled variance} = \frac{99 \times 8.0 + 99 \times 14.0 + 99 \times 18.0}{297} = 13.333$$

$$\chi^2 = 297 \times \ln 13.333 - 99 \times \ln 8.0 - 99 \times \ln 14.0 - 99 \times \ln 18.0$$
$$= 297 \times 2.58776 - 99 \times 2.079 - 99 \times 2.639 - 99 \times 2.890$$
$$= 768.58 - 753.19$$
$$= 15.37$$

We have three separate groups, and, so, $3-1 = 2$ degrees of freedom. The Chi-square table (Chap. 4) shows that a significant difference between the three variances is demonstrated at $p < 0.001$. If the three groups are representative comparable samples, we may conclude that these three insulin regimens do not produce the same spread of glucose levels.

Notes

An alternative to the Bartlett's test is the Levene's test. The Levene's test is less sensitive than the Bartlett's test to departures from normality. If there is a strong evidence that the data do in fact come from a normal, or nearly normal, distribution, then Bartlett's test has a better performance. Levene's test requires a lot of arithmetic, and is usually performed using statistical software. E.g., it is routinely used by SPSS when performing an unpaired t-test or one way ANOVA (analysis of variance) (see also Cleophas, Zwinderman, SPSS for Starters, part 1, Springer New York, 2010, Chaps. 4 and 8).

We should add that assessing significance of differences between 3 or more variances does not answer which of the samples produced the best outcome. Just like with analysis of variance, separate post hoc one by one analyses are required.

Conclusion

In some clinical studies the spread of the data may be more relevant than the average of the data. For example, the spread of glucose levels of a slow-release insulin may be more important than average values. In part I of this title, Chapter 16, the chi-square testing variability for one sample and the F-test for two samples have been explained. In this chapter the Bartlett's test, suitable for comparing two or more samples, is explained.

Chapter 16
Binary Partitioning for CART (Classification and Regression Tree) Methods

Binary partitioning is used to determine the best fit decision cut-off levels for a dataset with false positive and false negative patients. It serves a purpose similar to that of the receiver operating characteristic (ROC) curve method (Cleophas and Zwinderman, SPSS for Starters, Part 1, Chap. 17, Springer, New York, 2010), but, unlike ROC curves, it is adjusted for the magnitude of the samples, and therefore more precise. A hypothesized example is given in Fig. 16.1.

With binary partitioning, otherwise called the entropy method or classification and regression tree (CART) method, the entire sample of patients (Fig. 16.1) is called the parent node, which can, subsequently, be repeatedly split, partitioned if you will, into binary internal nodes. Mostly, internal nodes contain false positive or negative patients, and are, thus, somewhat impure. The magnitude of their impurity is assessed by the log likelihood method (see Chap. 13, part 1 of this title). Impurity equals the maximum log likelihood of the y-axis-variable by assuming that the x-axis-variable follows a Gaussian (i.e. binomial) distribution and is expressed in units, sometimes called bits (a short-cut for "binary digits"). All this sounds rather complex, but it works smoothly.

$$\text{The x-axis variable for the right node} = x_r = a/(a+b),$$
$$\text{for the left node} = x_l = d/(d+c).$$

If the impurity equals 1.0 bits, then it is maximal, if it equals 0.0, then it is minimal.

$$\text{Impurity node either right or left} = -x \ln x - (1-x)(1-x)\ln(1-x),$$

where ln means natural logarithm.

The impurities of the right and left node are calculated separately. Then, a weighted overall impurity of each cut-off level situation is calculated according to (* = sign of multiplication):

T. J. Cleophas and A. H. Zwinderman, *Statistical Analysis of Clinical Data on a Pocket Calculator, Part 2*, SpringerBriefs in Statistics, DOI: 10.1007/978-94-007-4704-3_16,
© The Author(s) 2012

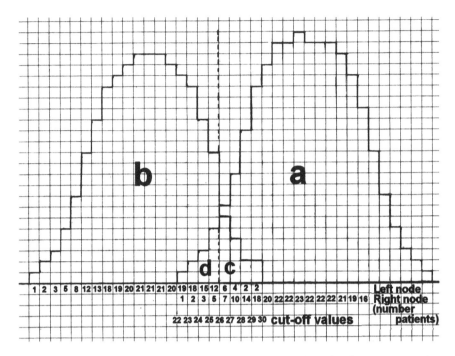

Fig. 16.1 Histogram of a patients' sample assessed for peripheral vascular disease; **a** summarizes the patients with a positive test and the presence of disease, **b** the patients with a negative test and the absence of disease, **c** and **d** are the false positive and false negative patients respectively

$$\text{Weighted impurity cut-off} = [(a + b)/(a + b + c + d) * \text{impurity-right-node}]$$
$$+ [(d + c)/(a + b + c + d) * \text{impurity-left-node}].$$

Underneath, an overview is given of the calculated impurities at the different cut-off levels. The cut-off percentage of 27 gives the smallest weighted impurity, and is, thus, the best fit predictor for the presence of peripheral vascular disease.

Cut-off (%)	Impurity right node	Impurity left node	Impurity weighted
22	0.5137	0.0000	0.3180
23	0.4392	0.0559	0.3063
24	0.4053	0.0982	0.2766
25	0.3468	0.1352	0.2711
26	0.1988	0.1688	0.1897
27	**0.1352**	**0.2268**	**0.1830**
28	0.0559	0.3025	0.1850
29	0.0559	0.3850	0.2375
30	0.0000	0.4690	0.2748

From the above calculation it can be concluded that a cut-off of 27 % is the best fit decision cut-off level with fewest false positive and fewest false negative patients. The result was slightly different from that of the ROC curve analysis, which produced a cut-off level of 26 %.

Conclusion

Binary partitioning is used to determine the best fit decision cut-off levels for a dataset with false positive and false negative patients. It serves a purpose similar to that of the receiver operating characteristic (ROC) curve method (Cleophas and Zwinderman. SPSS for Starters. Part I, Chapter 17. Springer. New York, 2010). but. unlike ROC curves. it is adjusted for the magnitude of the samples, and therefore more precise. The methodology is explained.

Chapter 17
Meta-Analysis of Continuous Data

Meta-analyses can be defined as systematic reviews with pooled data. Because the separate studies in a meta-analysis have different sample sizes, for the overall results a weighted average has to be calculated. Heterogeneity in a meta-analysis means that the differences in the results between the studies are larger than could happen by chance. The calculation of the overall result and the test for heterogeneity is demonstrated underneath.

Example

A meta-analysis of the difference in systolic blood pressures (mm Hg) between patients treated with potassium and those with placebo. Difference = difference in systolic blood pressure between patients on potassium and placebo, variance = (standard error)^2

	N	Difference (systolic)	Standard error	1/ variance	Difference/ variance	Difference^2/ variance
1. McGregor 1982	23	−7.0	3.1	0.104	−0.728	5.096
2. Siani 1987	37	−14.0	4.0	0.063	−0.875	12.348
3. Svetkey 1987	101	−6.4	1.9	0.272	−1.773	11.346
4. Krishna 1989	10	−5.5	3.8	0.069	−0.380	2.087
5. Obel 1989	48	−41.0	2.6	0.148	−6.065	248.788

(continued)

T. J. Cleophas and A. H. Zwinderman, *Statistical Analysis of Clinical Data on a Pocket Calculator, Part 2*, SpringerBriefs in Statistics, DOI: 10.1007/978-94-007-4704-3_17,
© The Author(s) 2012

(continued)

	N	Difference (systolic)	Standard error	1/ variance	Difference/ variance	Difference^2/ variance
6. Patki 1990	37	−12.1	2.6	0.148	−1.791	21.669
7. Fotherby 1992	18	−10.0	3.8	0.069	−0.693	6.900
8. Brancati 1996	87	−6.9	1.2	0.694	−4.792	33.041
9. Gu 2001	150	−5.0	1.4	0.510	−2.551	12.750
10. Sarkkinen 2011	45	−11.3	4.8	0.043	−0.490	5.091
				2.125	−20.138	359.516

Pooled difference = −20.138/2.125 = −9.48 mm Hg
Chi-square value for pooled data = (−20.138)^2/2.125 = 206.91
According to the Chi-square table (see Chap. 4) the p-value for 1 degree of freedom = <0.001

Heterogeneity of this meta-analysis is tested by the fixed effect model.
Heterogeneity chi-square value = 359.516 − 206.91 = 152.6,
With 9 degrees of freedom the p-value   = <0.001.

Although the meta-analysis shows a significantly lower systolic blood pressure in patients with potassium treatment than those with placebo, this result has a limited meaning, since the studies are significantly heterogeneous. For heterogeneity testing it is tested whether there is a greater inequalities between the results of the separate trials than is compatible with the play of chance. Additional tests for heterogeneity testing are available (Cleophas and Zwinderman, Meta-analysis. In: Statistics Applied to Clinical Studies, Springer New York, 2012, 5th edition, pp 365–388). However, when there is heterogeneity, a careful investigation of its potential cause is often more important than a lot of additional statistical tests.

Conclusion

Because the separate studies in a meta-analysis have different sample sizes for the overall results a weighted average has to be calculated. Heterogeneity in a meta-analysis means that the differences in the results between the studies are larger than could happen by chance. The calculation of the overall result and the test for heterogeneity is demonstrated.

Chapter 18
Meta-Analysis of Binary Data

Meta-analyses can be defined as systematic reviews with pooled data. Because the separate studies in a meta-analysis have different sample sizes for the overall results a weighted average has to be calculated. Heterogeneity in a meta-analysis means that the differences in the results between the studies are larger than could happen by chance. The calculation of the overall result and the test for heterogeneity is demonstrated underneath.

Example

The underneath data show the results of seven studies assessing chance of death and infarction in patients with coronary collaterals compared to that in patients without.

	Odds collaterals p	Odds no collaterals	n	Odds ratio	95 % ci		Z-value
Monteiro 2003	6/29	11/24	70	0.45	0.15–1.40	−1.38	1.69
Nathou 2006	3/173	20/365	561	0.32	0.09–1.08	−1.84	0.066
Meier 2007	36/190	197/389	812	0.37	0.25–0.56	−4.87	0.0001
Sorajja 2007	7/112	15/184	318	0.77	0.30–1.94	−0.56	0.576
Regieli 2009	7/254	16/600	879	1.03	0.42–2.54	+0.07	0.944
Desch 2010	5/64	34/132	235	0.30	0.11–0.81	−2.38	0.018
Steg 2010	246/1676	42/209	2173	0.73	0.51–1.04	−1.72	0.085

In order to meta-analyze these data, the following calculations are required. OR = odds ratio, ln OR = the natural logarithm of the odds ratio, var = variance.

T. J. Cleophas and A. H. Zwinderman, *Statistical Analysis of Clinical Data on a Pocket Calculator, Part 2*, SpringerBriefs in Statistics, DOI: 10.1007/978-94-007-4704-3_18, © The Author(s) 2012

	OR	ln OR	var	1/var	lnOR/var	$(\ln OR)^2$/var
Monteiro 2003	0.45	−0.795	0.3337	2.997	−2.382	1.894
Nathou 2006	0.32	−1.150	0.3919	2.882	−2.935	3.375
Meier 2007	0.37	−0.983	0.04069	24.576	−24.158	23.748
Sorajja 2007	0.77	−0.266	0.2239	4.466	−1.188	0.3160
Regieli 2009	1.03	−1.194	0.2526	3.959	−4.727	5.644
Desch 2010	0.30	0.032	0.2110	4.739	0.152	0.005
Steg 2010	0.73	−0.314	0.0333	30.03	9.429	2.961
				73.319	−44.667	37.943

The pooled odds ratio is calculated from antiln of $(-44.667/73.319) = 0.54$ (see Chap. 2 for the antiln (anti-logaritm) calculation).

The Chi-square value for pooled data $= (-44.667)^2/73.319 = 27.2117$

According to the Chi-square table (see Chap. 4) the p-value for 1 degree of freedom $= < 0.001$

Heterogeneity of this meta-analysis is tested by the fixed effect model.

Heterogeneity Chi-square value $= 37.943 - 27.2117$

$$= 10.7317$$

With 6 degrees of freedom the p-value $= 0.05 < p < 0.10$

Although the meta-analysis shows a significantly lower risk in patients with collaterals than in those without, this result has a limited meaning, since there is a trend to a significant heterogeneity. For heterogeneity testing it is tested whether the differences between the results of the separate trials are greater than compatible with the play of chance. Additional tests for heterogeneity testing are available (Cleophas and Zwinderman, Meta-analysis. In: Statistics Applied to Clinical Studies, Springer New York, 2012, 5th edition, pp 365–388). However, when there is heterogeneity, a careful investigation of its potential cause is often more important than a lot of additional statistical tests.

Conclusion

Because the separate studies in a meta-analysis have different sample sizes for the overall results a weighted average has to be calculated. Heterogeneity in a meta-analysis means that the differences in the results between the studies are larger than could happen by chance. The calculation of the overall result and the test for heterogeneity is demonstrated.

Chapter 19
Physicians' Daily Life and the Scientific Method

We assumed the numbers of unanswered questions in the physicians' daily life would be large. But just to get an impression, one of the authors of this chapter (TC) recorded all of the unanswered answers he asked himself during a single busy day. Excluding the questions with uncertain but generally accepted answers, he included 9 questions.

During the hospital rounds 8.00–12.00 h.

1. Do I continue, stop or change antibiotics with fever relapse after 7 days treatment?
2. Do I prescribe a secondary prevention of a venous thrombosis for 3, 6 months or permanently?
3. Should I stop anticoagulant treatment or continue with a hemorrhagic complication in a patient with an acute lung embolia?
4. Is the rise in falling out of bed lately real or due to chance?
5. Do I perform a liver biopsy or wait and see with liver function disturbance without obvious cause?

During the outpatient clinic 13.00–17.00 h.

6. Do I prescribe aspirin, hydroxy-carbamide or wait and see in a patient with a thrombocytosis of $800 \times 10^{12}/l$ over 6 months?
7. Are fundic gland polyps much more common in females than in males?

During the staff meeting 17.00–18.00 h

8. Is the large number of physicians with burn out due to chance or the result of a local problem?
9. Is the rise in patients' letters of complaints a chance effect or a real effect to worry about?

T. J. Cleophas and A. H. Zwinderman, *Statistical Analysis of Clinical Data on a Pocket Calculator, Part 2*, SpringerBriefs in Statistics, DOI: 10.1007/978-94-007-4704-3_19, © The Author(s) 2012

Many of the above questions did not qualify for a simple statistical assessment, but others did. The actual assessments, that were very clarifying for our purposes, are given underneath.

Falling Out of Bed

If more patients fall out of bed than expected, a hospital department will put much energy in finding the cause and providing better prevention. If, however, the scores tend to rise, another approach is to first assess whether or not the rise is due to chance, because daily life is full of variations. To do so the numbers of events observed is compared to the numbers of event in a sister department. The pocket calculator method is a straightforward method for that purpose.

	Patients with fall out of bed	Patients without	
Department 1	16 (a)	26 (b)	42 (a + b)
Department 2	5 (c)	30 (d)	35 (c + d)
	21 (a + c)	56 (b + d)	77 (a + b + c + d)

Pocket calculator method:

$$\text{chi} - \text{square} \quad = \quad \frac{(ad - bc)^2 (a + b + c + d)}{(a + b)(c + d)(b + d)(a + c)} \quad = \quad 5.456$$

If the Chi-square (Chi-square table Chap. 15) value is larger than 3.841, then a statistically significant difference between the two departments will be accepted at $p < 0.05$. This would mean that in this example, indeed, the difference is larger than could be expected by chance and that a further examination of the measures to prevent fall out of bed is warranted.

Evaluation of Fundic Gland Polyps

A physician has the impression that fundic gland polyps are more common in females than it is in males. Instead of reporting this subjective finding, he decides to follow the next two months every patient in his program.

	Patients with fundic gland polyps	Patients without	
Females	15 (a)	20 (b)	35 (a + b)
Males	15 (c)	5 (d)	20 (c + d)
	30 (a + c)	25 (b + d)	55 (a + b + c + d)

Pocket calculator method:

$$chi - square = \frac{(ad - bc)^2(a + b + c + d)}{(ab)(c + d)(b + d)(a + c)} = 5.304$$

The calculated Chi-square value is again larger than 3.841. The difference between males and females is significant at p < 0.05. We can be for about 95 % sure that the difference between the genders is real and not due to chance. The physician can report to his colleagues that the difference in genders is to be taken into account in future work-ups.

Physicians with a Burn-Out

Two partnerships of specialists have the intention to associate. However, during meetings, it was communicated that in one of the two partnerships there were three specialists with burn-out. The meeting decided not to consider this as chance finding, but requested a statistical analysis of this finding under the assumption that unknown factors in partnership one may place these specialists at an increased risk of a burn-out.

	Physicians with burn out	Without burn out	
Partnership 1	3 (a)	7 (b)	10 (a + b)
Partnership 2	0 (c)	10 (d)	10 (c + d)
	3 (a + c)	17(b + d)	20 (a + b + c + d)

Pocket calculator method

$$chi - square = \frac{(ad - bc)^2(a + b + c + d)}{(a + b)(c + d)(b + d)(a + c)} = \frac{(30 - 0)2(20)}{10 \times 10 \times 17 \times 3}$$
$$= \frac{900 \times 20}{\dots} = 3.6$$

The Chi-square value was between 2.706 and 3.841. This means that no significant difference between the two partnerships exists, but there is a trend to a difference at p < 0.10. This was communicated back to the meeting and it was decided to disregard the trend. Ten years later no further case of burn-out had been observed.

Patients'Letters of Complaints

In a hospital the number of patients' letters of complaints was twice the number in the period before. The management was deeply worried and issued an in-depth analysis of possible causes. One junior manager recommended that prior to this laborious exercise it might be wise to first test whether the increase might be due to chance rather than a real effect.

	Patients with letter of complaints	Patients without	
year 2006	10 (a)	1000 (b)	1010 (a + b)
year 2005	5 (c)	1000 (d)	1005 (c + d)
	15 (a + c)	2000 (b + d)	2015 (a + b + c + d)

$$\text{chi} - \text{square} = \frac{(ad - bc)^2(a + b + c + d)}{(a + b)(c + d)(b + d)(a + c)} = 1.64..$$

The Chi-square was smaller than 2.706, and so the difference could not be ascribed to any effect to worry about but rather to chance. No further analysis of the differences between 2006 and 2005 were performed.

There are, of course, many questions in physicians' daily life that are less straightforward and cannot be readily answered at the workplace with a pocket calculator. E.g., the effects of subgroups and other covariates in a patient group will require t-tests, analyses of variance, likelihood ratio tests, and regression models. Fortunately, in the past 15 years user-friendly statistical software and self-assessment programs have been developed that can help answering complex questions. The complementary titles of this book, entitled SPSS for Starters part 1 and 2 from the same authors, are helpful for the purpose.

Conclusion

Few physicians have followed the scientific method for answering practical questions they simply do not know the answer to. The scientific method is in a nutshell: reformulate your question into a hypothesis and try and test this hypothesis against control observations. Simple examples are given.

Chapter 20
Incident Analysis and the Scientific Method

The PRISMA (Prevention and Recovery System for Monitoring and Analysis)-, CIA (Critical Incident Analysis)-, CIT (Critical Incident Technique)-, TRIPOD (tripod-theory based method)—methods are modern approaches to incident— analysis. It is unclear why the scientific method has been systematically ignored in incident—analysis.

Example

As example the case of a fatal hemorrhage in a hospital during an observational period of one year was used. In case of a fatal hemorrhage the physician in charge of the analysis will first make an inventory of how many fatal hemorrhages of the same kind have occurred in the period of one year. The number seems to be ten.

The null—hypothesis is that 0 hemorrhages will occur per year, and the question is whether 10 is significantly more than 0. A one—sample—z-test is used.

$$z = \text{(mean number)} / \text{(standard error)} = 10/\sqrt{10} = 3.16.$$
z - value is larger than 3.080 (see z-table, Chap. 2).
p - value is <0.002.

The number 10 is, thus, much larger than a number that could occur by accident (see z-table, Chap. 2). Here an avoidable error could very well be responsible. However, a null—hypothesis of 0 hemorrhages is probably not correct, because a year without fatal hemorrhages, actually, never happens. Therefore, we will compare the number of fatal hemorrhages in the given year with that of the year before. There were five fatal hemorrhages then. The z-test produces the following result (see z-table Chap. 2).

T. J. Cleophas and A. H. Zwinderman, *Statistical Analysis of Clinical Data on a Pocket Calculator, Part 2*, SpringerBriefs in Statistics, DOI: 10.1007/978-94-007-4704-3_20, © The Author(s) 2012

Table 20.1 Rates of fatal hemorrhages in a hospital during two subsequent year of observation. According to the chi-square statistic <3.84 the difference in rates is not significant

	Year 1	Year 2
Number fatal hemorrhages	10	5
Number control patients	9990	9995

$$\text{Chi} - \text{square} = \frac{(10 \times 9995 + 5 \times 9990)^2 (20000)}{10 \times 9990 \times 5 \times 9995} = 1.62$$

Table 20.2 Log likelihood ratio test of the data from Table 20.1. Also this test is not significant with a Chi-square value smaller than 3.84

$$\text{Log likelihood ratio} = 5 \log \frac{(10/9990)}{5/9995} + 9995 \frac{\log(1 - 10/9990)}{1 - 5/9995}$$

$$= 3.468200 - 5.008856 = -1.540656$$

$$\text{Chi} - \text{square} = -2 \log - \text{likelihood} - \text{ratio} = 3.0813$$

log natural logarithm

$$z = (10 - 5) / \sqrt{(10 + 5)} = 1.29$$

$$\text{p - value} = \text{not significant because z is} < 1.96.$$

We can, however, question whether both years are representative for a longer period of time. Epidemiological data have established that an incident-reduction of 70 % is possible with optimal quality health care. We test whether 10 is significantly different from $(10-(70\%) \times 10) = 3$. The z-test shows the following (z table Chap. 2).

$$z = (10 - 3) / \sqrt{(10 + 3)} = 1.94$$

$$\text{p - value} = 0.05 < \text{p} < 0.10$$

It means that here also no significant effect has been demonstrated. A more sensitive mode of testing will be obtained, if we take into account the entire number of admissions per year. In the given hospital there were 10,000 admissions in either of the two years. A Chi-square test can now be performed according to the 2×2 contingency table in Table 20.1. With one degree of freedom this value ought to have been at least 3.84 in order to demonstrate whether a significant difference is in the data (Chi-square table Chap. 4). And, so, again there is no significant difference between the two years.

Finally, a log—likelihood—ratio - test is performed, a test which falls into the category of exact—tests, and is, therefore, still somewhat more sensitive (see also Chap. 13 of the part 1 of this title). The result is in Table 20.2. It is close to 3.84, but still somewhat smaller. Also this test shows no significant difference between the frequencies of deadly fatal hemorrhages in the two years of observation.

The analyst in charge takes the decision to perform one last test, making use of epidemiological data that have shown that with optimal health care quality in a facility similar to ours we may accept with 95 % confidence that the number of

Example   71

fatal hemorrhages will remain below 20 per 10,000 admissions. With 10 deadly bleedings the 95 % confidence interval can be calculated to be 5-18 (calculated from the Internet "Confidence interval calculator for proportions", http://faculty.vassar.edu). This result is under 20. Also from this analysis it can be concluded that a profound research of the fatal hemorrhages is not warranted. The number of hemorrhages falls under the boundary of optimal quality care.

The scientific method is often defined as an evaluation of clinical data based on appropriate statistical tests, rather than a description of the cases and their summaries. The above example explains that the scientific method can be helpful in giving a clue to which incidents are based on randomness and which are not so.

Conclusion

Many software progams provide a systematic approach to the explanation of a single incident at the workplace. Few programs have followed the scientific method for assessing causal relationships between factors and the resulting incident. The scientific method is in a nutshell: reformulate your question into a hypothesis and try and test this hypothesis against control observations. Examples are given.

Final Remarks

Clinical studies often assess the efficacy of new treatments/treatment modalities.

The first part of this issue reviewed basic statistical analysis methods. There are, however, many questions in clinical studies that are not answered by the simple tests, and additional methodologies are required.

Particularly, methods for dealing with imperfect data and outliers are an important objective of part 2 of this issue, the current e book. Many of these methods are computationally intensive, and require statistical software. But, fortunately, others can be conveniently carried out on scientific pocket calculator.

Apart from methodologies for assessing imperfect data and data outliers (Chaps. 3–7), attention is given to tests that are helpful to improve your research like the item response modeling and superiority testing (Chaps. 13–15). The basic statistical analysis of meta-analysis is not complex, and weighting procedures and heterogeneity assessment of meta-analyses are given in the Chaps. 17 and 18. Finally, simple tests for incident analysis and the analysis of unexpected observations at the workplace are reviewed in the Chaps. 19 and 20.

The advantage of the pocket calculator is that:

1. You better understand what you are doing. The statistical software program is kind of black box program.
2. The pocket calculator works faster, because far less steps have to be taken.
3. The pocket calculator works faster, because averages can be used.
4. With statistical software all individual data have to be included separately, a time-consuming activity in case of large data files.

Also pocket calculators are wonderful, because they enable you to test instantly at your workplace without the need to download a computer program.

T. J. Cleophas and A. H. Zwinderman, *Statistical Analysis of Clinical Data on a Pocket Calculator, Part 2*, SpringerBriefs in Statistics, DOI: 10.1007/978-94-007-4704-3,

Additional reasons for writing this e book are the following.

1. To review the basic principles of statistical testing which tends to be increasingly forgotten in the current computer era.
2. To serve as a primer for nervous investigators who would like to perform their own data analyses but feel inexpert to do so.
3. To make investigators better understand what they are doing, when analyzing clinical data.
4. To facilitate data analysis by use of a number of *rapid* pocket calculator methods.
5. As a primer for those who wish to master more advanced statistical methods. More advanced methods are reviewed by the same authors in the books "SPSS for Starters, Part 1 and part 2" 2010 and 2012, "Statistics Applied to Clinical Studies" 5th edition, 2012, "Statistics Applied to Clinical Trials: Self-Assessment Book, 2002, all of them edited by Springer, Dordrecht. These books closely fit and complement the format and contents of the current e book.

Like the first part of this issue the current e book is very condensed, but this should be threshold lowering to readers. As a consequence, however, the theoretical background of the methods described are not sufficiently explained in the text. Extensive theoretical information is also given in the above mentioned books from the same authors.

Index

T. J. Cleophas and A. H. Zwinderman, *Statistical Analysis of Clinical Data on a Pocket Calculator, Part 2*, SpringerBriefs in Statistics, DOI: 10.1007/978-94-007-4704-3,
© The Author(s) 2012